Depression and Sleep

Depression
and Sleep

P J Cowen
MRC Clinical Scientist,
Littlemore Hospital,
Oxford OX4 4XN

MARTIN DUNITZ

First published in the United Kingdom
in 1997 by
Martin Dunitz Ltd
The Livery House
7– 9 Pratt Street
London NW1 0AE

A CIP record for this book is available
from the British Library.

ISBN 1-85317-358-4

Printed and bound in Spain by Cayfosa

Contents

Normal sleep

Humans spend about one third of their lives asleep but despite intensive research the physiological function of sleep remains obscure. Sleep can be defined as a periodic state of rest, characterized by loss of conscious awareness, quiescence of physiological functions and reduced responsiveness to external stimuli.

Pattern of sleep

Sleep is in essence a behavioural state, but measurements of brain electrical activity by electroencephalography (EEG) show characteristic changes in pattern over the sleep period. There are two major kinds of sleep. The first is *quiet, synchronized* or non-rapid eye movement (NREM) sleep and the second is known variously as *desynchronized, paradoxical, rapid eye movement (REM)* or *dream* sleep. Generally, over the night an individual will experience four or five cycles of quiet sleep alternating with REM sleep; however, REM sleep becomes more prominent during the latter part of the sleep period.

Quiet sleep

Quiet sleep is itself divided into stages which correspond to increased depth of sleep, with progressive relaxation of the muscles, and increasing arousal threshold. These stages were defined by Rechtschaffen and Kales[1] according to their characteristic EEG appearance. Sleep stages are scored in small segments (usually of about 30 seconds) which are known as epochs.

- **Wake**. In relaxed wakefulness with the eyes closed the EEG is characterized by alpha waves (8–12 cycles/second) and low-voltage activity of mixed frequency. Eye movements are often present and the muscle tone or electromyogram activity (EMG) is usually high. As the subject becomes drowsy, alpha waves diminish and the eyes may begin to roll (Figure 1).

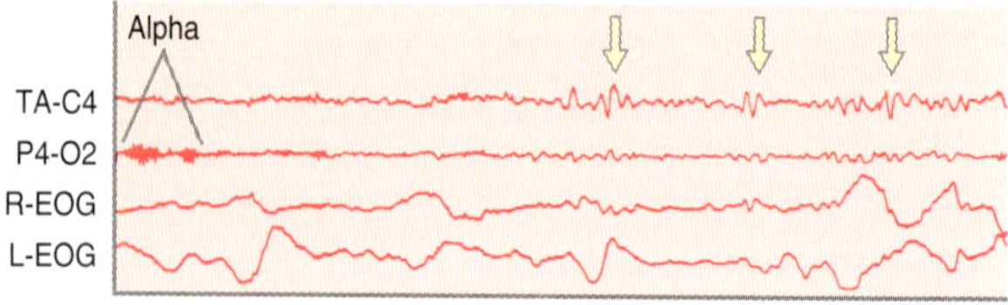

Figure 1
Sleep EEG recording of relaxed wakefulness and stage 1 sleep, showing EEG leads (T4-C4; P4-O2) and eye movements (EOG). Arrows indicate vertex sharp waves (reproduced from reference[1] with permission of Wrightson Biomedical Publishing Ltd, Petersfield, 1991).

- **Stage 1**. This is the lightest stage of sleep and is regarded as transitional between sleep and wakefulness. Alpha waves decrease to less than 50% of the EEG record. Vertex sharp waves may be present. Rolling eye movements are present and EMG activity is decreased. Stage 1 in normal sleep is of short duration (about 1–7 minutes) (Figure 1).

- **Stage 2**. In stage 2 sleep the EEG background is largely of theta waves which have a frequency of 3.5–7.5 cycles/second. Also present are K complexes (a negative wave followed 0.75 seconds later by a positive wave) and sleep spindles which are brief bursts of waves of 12–14 cycles/second lasting at least 0.5 seconds (Figure 2).

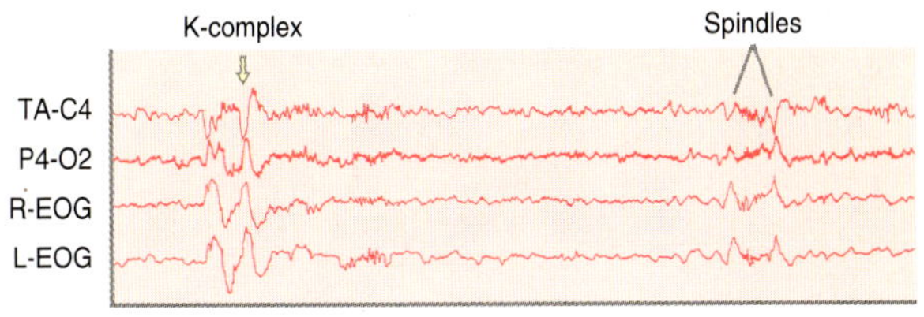

Figure 2
Sleep EEG recording of stage 2 sleep (reproduced from reference[1] with permission of Wrightson Biomedical Publishing Ltd, Petersfield, 1991).

- **Stage 3**. This is characterized by the appearance of delta waves which have a high amplitude (>75 μv) and low frequency (<3.5 cycles/second). To qualify as stage 3 the record must contain between 20 and 50% delta waves. Sleep spindles sometimes persist into stage 3 sleep (Figure 3).

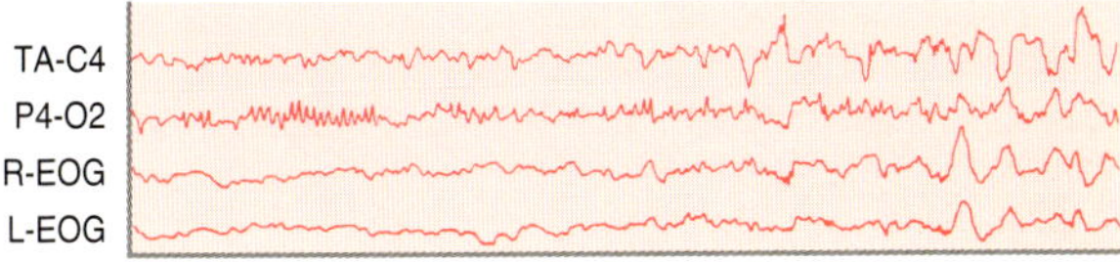

Figure 3
Sleep EEG recording of stage 3 sleep with delta waves at the end of the record (reproduced from reference[1] with permission of Wrightson Biomedical Publishing Ltd, Petersfield, 1991).

- **Stage 4**. This is dominated by delta waves which make up more than 50% of the record. As with stage 3 sleep, sleep spindles may be present. Often, in sleep EEG studies, stages 3 and 4 sleep are combined to give a measurement of total *slow wave* or *deep* sleep (Figure 4).

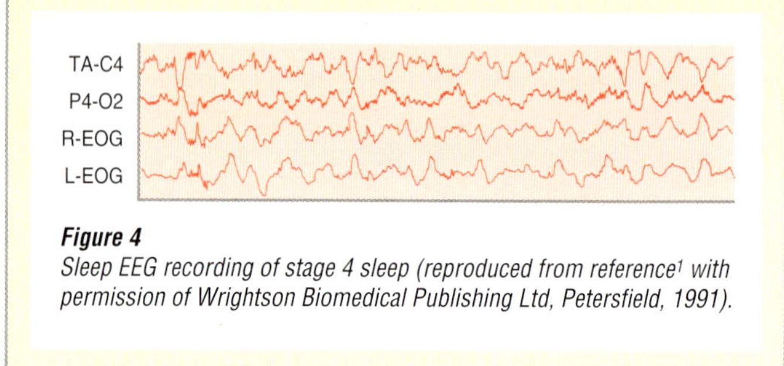

Figure 4
Sleep EEG recording of stage 4 sleep (reproduced from reference[1] with permission of Wrightson Biomedical Publishing Ltd, Petersfield, 1991).

REM sleep

The classification of the EEG into sleep stages by sleep records is a somewhat arbitrary division of a continuous process. More importantly, quiet sleep is interrupted by four or five periods of a different form of sleep that has some EEG resemblance to stage 1 and wake. Persons awakened during these periods frequently report dreaming. The four or five periods of REM or dream sleep that occur during the night take up a total time of about 90 minutes, a little more than 20% of total sleep time (Table 1) .

Stage 1	2–5%
Stage 2	45–55%
Stage 3	3–8%
Stage 4	10–15%
NREM (stages 1+2+3+4)	75–80%
REM sleep	20–25%
Wakefulness	~5%

Table 1
Different stages of sleep in a normal young adult.

In the EEG, REM sleep is characterized by low-voltage, mixed frequency activity with episodic, jerky, horizontal, vertical and oblique conjugate rapid eye movements. The presence of saw-tooth waves can help distinguish REM sleep from stage 1 sleep. EMG activity reaches its lowest level and may be accompanied by phasic muscle twitches (Figure 5); K complexes and sleep spindles are absent. Autonomic changes are also apparent in REM sleep, including irregularity in pulse rate, respiratory rate and blood pressure, and penile erections in the male.

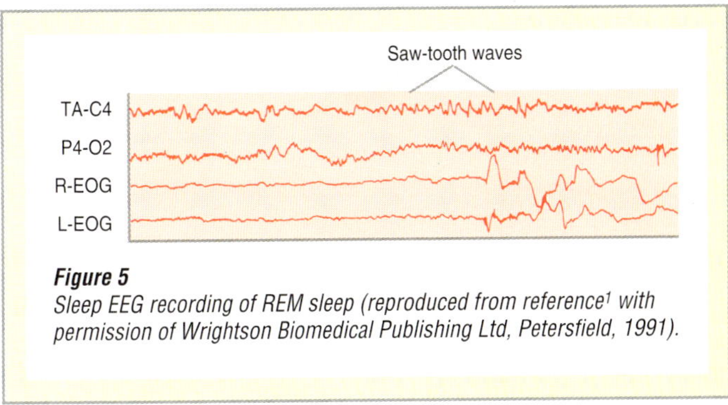

Figure 5
Sleep EEG recording of REM sleep (reproduced from reference[1] with permission of Wrightson Biomedical Publishing Ltd, Petersfield, 1991).

The sleep hypnogram

The cyclical pattern of sleep during the night is often plotted as a sleep hypnogram (Figure 6). A young adult passes from waking into quiet sleep and it is about 70–90 minutes before the first period of REM sleep occurs. This is called the REM latency. Stage 2 has a pivotal role in sleep organization in that it is involved in all stage transitions other than that between 3 and 4. Over the night the amount of slow wave sleep decreases while that of REM sleep increases. Each cycle of sleep in a young adult takes about 90 minutes.

Changes over the life cycle

A new-born child sleeps 16–18 hours daily and about half of this is REM sleep. A young adult spends 16–17 hours awake

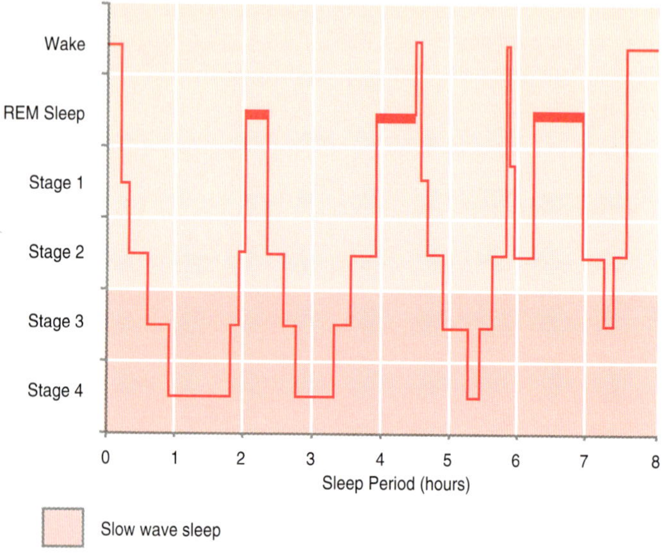

Figure 6
Sleep hypnogram in a healthy young adult.

and 7–8 hours asleep, of which perhaps about 6 hours consist of quiet sleep with an additional 1.5 hours of REM sleep. The elderly tend to sleep less at night although they are more likely to take daytime naps. During sleep the elderly experience more awakenings and have less stage 4 sleep.

Sleep continuity and efficiency

Normal subjects have several short awakenings during the night, but unless these last more than about 2 minutes they are not consciously experienced. Subjects who report awareness of multiple awakenings often experience their sleep as unre-freshing. Measures of sleep continuity in the EEG therefore provide important information about how sleep is likely to be experienced. Such measures include the time taken to fall asleep, the total time spent awake after initially falling asleep and the time of final awakening. Another important measure is that of *sleep efficiency* which is calculated as the percentage of time in bed an individual actually spends asleep. In healthy young subjects, sleep efficiency is usually about 90% or more.

Functions of sleep

All mammals sleep and all have periods of both quiet and REM sleep, with the exception of dolphins who do not appear to have REM sleep, perhaps because they need to swim continuously. Because REM sleep and quiet sleep are so different physiologically, it has been argued that they probably subserve different functions in both humans and other animals.[2]

REM sleep

A striking phenomenon of REM sleep is its high prevalence in neonates and young children. This has given rise to suggestions that it may be involved in brain development, perhaps in providing a high level of cerebral stimulation. Other suggestions are that it provides alternative strategies for problem solving or helps to eliminate spurious connections in neuronal networks accumulated during the day. It is worth noting that selective REM sleep deprivation in healthy adult humans produces little detectable change in psychological well-being.

Slow wave sleep

There is some evidence that slow wave sleep is important for what is loosely termed *cerebral restitution*. Sleep deprivation has more striking effects on cerebral function than that of other tissues. This may be because during wake the cerebrum retains a state of constant alertness and sleep, particularly the deeper stages, may provide an opportunity for consolidation of neuronal networks and synaptic repair. In small rodents, sleep may enable energy conservation but this is unlikely to play an important role in humans.

Sleep disorders

Epidemiology

Complaints of insomnia are common, particularly in the middle-aged and elderly.[3] About one in four Americans complain of occasional insomnia while almost 10% have regular, long-standing sleep difficulties. People with insomnia complain that sleep is unrefreshing and they wake feeling particularly drowsy and tired. The most common reported problem is waking during the night with difficulty falling asleep again. This can be demonstrated in the sleep EEG as impaired sleep efficiency, which is defined as the percentage of time a person spends in bed that they are actually asleep (Table 2). It is worth noting that people with insomnia report a higher frequency of additional problems such as memory difficulty, impaired coping and poor interpersonal relationships

Sleep measure (mean)	Insomniacs	Controls
Time in bed (mins)	463	451
Actual sleep time (mins)	374	388
Sleep efficiency (%)	81*	86
Sleep onset latency (mins)	10	10
Wake after sleep onset (mins)	60*	33

* Significant difference from controls

Table 2
EEG measures of sleep continuity in 20 patients with primary insomnia and 20 healthy controls (from Attenburrow et al, unpublished).

Diagnosis

In the *Diagnostic and Statistical Manual of Mental Disorders* (DSM-IV),[4] primary sleep disorders are sleep problems that cannot be accounted for by another mental disorder, a general medical condition or substance use or withdrawal. Sleep disorders are subdivided into dyssomnias and parasomnias. Dyssomnias are characterized by abnormalities in the amount, quality or timing of sleep and would therefore include primary insomnia (Table 3). In contrast, parasomnias consist of abnormal behaviours or experiences occurring in association with sleep, specific sleep stages or sleep–wake transitions. For a review of these disorders, the reader should consult references 4 and 5.

(1) Dyssomnias	(a) Primary insomnia
	(b) Primary hypersomnia
	(c) Narcolepsy
	(d) Breathing-related sleep disorder (includes sleep apnoea)
	(e) Circadian rhythm sleep disorder (sleep-wake schedule disorder)
(2) Parasomnias	(a) Nightmare disorder
	(b) Sleep terror disorder
	(c) Sleepwalking disorder

Table 3
Primary sleep disorders in DSM-IV.

Treatment

The treatment of primary insomnia is often unsatisfactory. Non-drug treatments can include improved sleep hygiene, such as reducing total time spent in bed together with attention to the timing of meals and avoidance of caffeine-containing drinks.

Drug treatments such as benzodiazepines are helpful in the short term, but longer-term use is now well known to be associated with therapeutic tolerance and drug dependence. Most people with insomnia do not consult doctors about their sleep problems, but in the USA, about 40% of insomniacs medicate themselves with alcohol or over-the-counter hypnotics, usually sedating antihistamines. The long-term effects of this practice are uncertain.

The difficulty in treating primary insomnia makes it important to detect insomnia which occurs secondary to other causes. Sleep disorders are common in depressed patients and appropriate recognition and treatment of depression can successfully ameliorate both the depressive disorder and the associated insomnia.

Distributed neuronal networks particularly involving the brain stem reticular activating system, pons, thalamus and hypothalamus regulate the sleep–wake cycle and sleep architecture. The brain stem and midbrain contain the cell bodies of monoamine neurotransmitters such as noradrenaline, serotonin (5-HT), dopamine and acetylcholine. Drugs that alter the activity of these neurotransmitters can have striking effects on sleep and sleep architecture.[5,6]

5-HT pathways

The majority of the 5-HT-containing neurones of the brain stem are located in midline raphe nuclei. Destruction of the raphe nuclei in animals abolishes sleep. Similarly administration of the 5-HT synthesis inhibitor, para-chlorophenylalanine causes insomnia which can be reversed by the 5-HT precursor, 5-hydroxytryptophan. Raphe cells exhibit a regular firing pattern which is closely related to the level of consciousness. In the cat, for example, 5-HT cell firing is decreased during sleep and virtually ceases during REM sleep.[7]

The effects of 5-HT-altering drugs on human sleep do not fit a simple pattern, perhaps because of the multiplicity of 5-HT receptor subtypes, which have diverse functional roles. It is well established that drugs which selectively block the re-uptake of 5-HT lower REM sleep and increase wakefulness. However, the same is seen with the 5-HT synthesis inhibitor, parachlorophenylalanine.

There is more consistent evidence concerning the role of 5-HT_2 receptors in the regulation of slow wave sleep. For example, the selective 5-HT_2 receptor antagonist ritanserin produces a dose-related increase in slow wave sleep which persists with repeated treatment (Figure 7). The same is seen with less selective drugs that also have 5-HT_2 receptor antagonist properties such as mianserin and cyproheptadine. The 5-HT_2 receptor agonist m-chlorophenylpiperazine (mCPP) is a metabolite of the antidepressant drugs, trazodone and nefazodone. It produces a dose-related decrease in slow wave sleep and at higher doses also lowers REM sleep and decreases sleep continuity.[8]

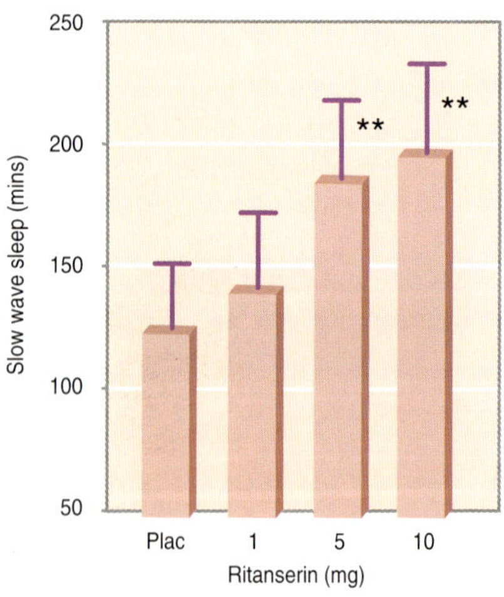

Figure 7
*The effect of single doses of the 5-HT₂ receptor antagonist ritanserin on sleep in healthy subjects (** denotes significantly greater than placebo).*

Noradrenaline

Noradrenaline cell bodies are located in the locus coeruleus. In animal studies stimulation of this brain region induces arousal and wakefulness. In both humans and animals, drugs that lower noradrenergic neurotransmission at post-synaptic α_1-adrenoceptors tend to cause sedation and increased sleep, while the reverse is the case for drugs that potentiate noradrenergic function.

Effects of noradrenergic drugs on REM sleep in humans are complex and do not conform to a simple pattern. For example, the α_2-adrenoceptor agonist clonidine lowers noradrenaline release by stimulating inhibitory cell body autoreceptors. As would be expected from this action clonidine causes sedation with decreased wake in the sleep EEG. Clonidine also decreases REM sleep. Paradoxically, however, the α_2-adrenoceptor antagonist idazoxan, a drug which increases noradrenaline release, also lowers REM sleep, although as expected it increases wake in the sleep EEG.[9]

The effects of α_1-adrenoceptor antagonists on REM sleep are rather unclear, perhaps because of the lack of specificity of the drugs used. However, the relatively selective α_1-adrenoceptor antagonist thymoxamine appears to increase REM sleep in humans. It is well recognized from clinical practice that lipophilic β-adrenoceptor antagonists can impair sleep. Propanolol, for example, increases wake and decreases REM sleep, although the reporting of vivid dreams is increased.

Dopamine

Drugs that indirectly increase post synaptic dopamine neurotransmission, such as amphetamine and pemoline, increase wakefulness and decrease sleep. Pemoline also decreases REM sleep but this may be because of the general decrease in overall sleep time.[9] On the other hand, the non-selective dopaminergic agent apomorphine decreases both REM sleep and slow wave sleep in humans without altering total sleep time.[10] In humans, dopamine receptor antagonists such as haloperidol produce little effect on either sleep architecture or sleep time.

Acetylcholine

There is good and consistent evidence from human and animal studies that acetylcholine pathways facilitate REM sleep. For example, the anticholinesterase drug physostigmine, which inhibits the metabolism of acetylcholine, hastens the onset of REM sleep. Interestingly, if infused during REM sleep it produces arousal. The muscarinic agonist arecholine also decreases REM latency if given during the first or second non-REM period. In contrast, muscarinic antagonists such as atropine delay the onset of REM sleep. Overall the data indicate that the muscarinic receptor activation plays a facilitatory role in the mediation of REM sleep.

Histamine

Histamine pathways originating from the midbrain are known to be involved in the regulation of arousal. Drugs that block histamine H_1-receptors, such as mepyramine, cause sedation and decrease wake in the sleep EEG. However, they do not have consistent effects on sleep architecture. In contrast, histamine H_2-receptor antagonists have little consistent effect on sleep or the sleep EEG, but cimetidine may increase slow wave sleep.

Gamma-aminobutyric acid

Gamma-aminobutyric acid (GABA) is the major inhibitory neurotransmitter in the brain. Facilitation of neurotransmission at GABA synapses causes sedation and has anticonvulsant effects. Benzodiazepines increase neurotransmission at GABA-A synapses by binding to a specific allosteric site on the post-synaptic GABA receptor complex. Benzodiazepines have prominent hypnotic effects and decrease wake in the sleep EEG. In addition, they change sleep architecture by decreasing REM and slow wave sleep and increasing stage 2 sleep. Newer hypnotics that facilitate GABA function, such as zolpidem and zopiclone, decrease wakefulness but have less effect on sleep architecture than benzodiazepines.[11]

Sleep in depression

Subjective complaints

Disturbed sleep is a characteristic symptom of depression. Patients may report several kinds of difficulty including delay in falling asleep, broken sleep and early morning waking, two or three hours before their usual time. After this, the patient does not fall asleep again but lies awake feeling unrefreshed and often restless and agitated. He thinks about the coming day with pessimism, broods about past failures and ponders gloomily about the future. It is this combination of early waking with depressive thinking that is important in diagnosis. Some patients, particularly those with bipolar depression or atypical depression, sleep excessively rather than wake early but they still find their sleep unrefreshing.

The experience of depressive sleep disturbance has been vividly described by William Styron:[12]

> "Exhaustion combined with sleeplessness is a rare torture... my few hours of sleep were terminated at three or four in the morning, when I stared up into yawning darkness, wondering and writhing at the devastation taking place in my mind and awaiting the dawn which usually permitted me a feverish, dreamless nap."

Sleep EEG in depression

Recordings of the sleep EEG in depressed patients have shown several abnormalities (Figure 8 and Table 4).[13,14] The most commonly found are:

- Impaired sleep and sleep continuity
- Decreased slow wave sleep
- Decreased latency to REM sleep
- An increase in the proportion of REM sleep in the early part of the night

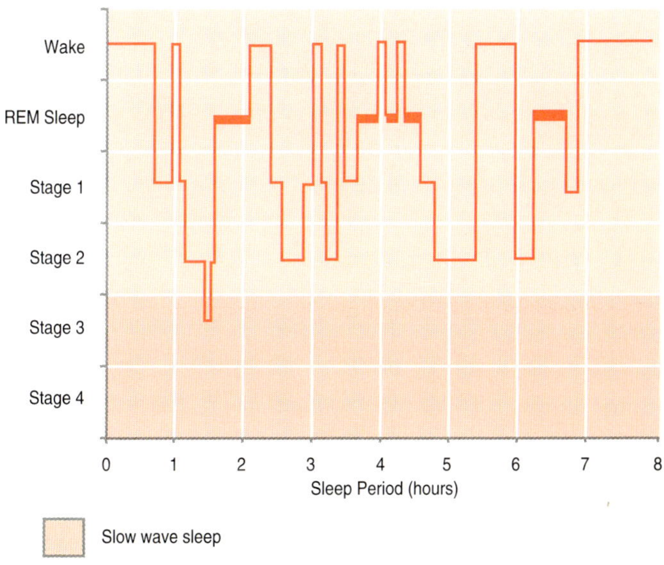

Figure 8
Sleep hypnogram in a depressed patient.

Sleep measure (mean)	Controls	Depressives
Actual sleep time (mins)	410	354*
Wake after sleep onset (mins)	20	30
Sleep efficiency (%)	92	84*
Sleep onset latency (mins)	17	34*
REM sleep (mins)	96	92
REM latency (mins)	87	52*
Slow wave sleep (%)	11	11

* Significant difference from controls.
Source: Thase et al[33]

Table 4
Sleep EEG measures in 20 depressed inpatients and 25 healthy controls.

REM latency

The decrease in REM latency has been a focus of particular research interest. There is some evidence that it may persist in recovered depressed patients and perhaps indicate a vulnerability to depressive relapse. Interestingly, first degree relatives of patients with depression may also exhibit decreased REM latency, even if they have never been depressed. A further link with depression is that many effective antidepressant drugs increase REM latency and decrease REM sleep time, although some newer agents, for example bupropion and nefazodone, do not.

Slow wave sleep

Depressed patients may also exhibit decreases in the amount of slow wave sleep in the sleep EEG. The decrease in slow wave sleep may persist after recovery, particularly in patients at high risk of a future recurrence.

Sleep continuity

The increased number of awakenings and decreased sleep efficiency commonly seen in depressed patients is associated with the subjective feeling of sleep being unrefreshing. Lessening of depression is associated with improvements in sleep continuity which leads to subjective benefit in the experience of sleep. In addition, resolution of depression with attendant negative cognitions is likely to improve the way in which patients perceive their sleep quality.

Antidepressant drugs can also influence sleep efficiency directly, independent of their effect on depressed mood. For example, sedating antidepressants can decrease awakenings and increase sleep efficiency. These useful effects, however, can be associated with day-time hangover (see Chapter 4).

Sleep deprivation and depression

The striking relationship between sleep and mood is illustrated by the acute antidepressant effect of sleep deprivation. Wu and Bunney[15] reviewed the published effects of one night of total sleep deprivation in 1700 depressed patients. On average 59% of subjects showed marked decreases in depressive symptoms the day following sleep deprivation. Response rates in patients with endogenous depression (67%) were higher than in those with neurotic depression (48%). Interestingly, repeated selective awakenings of depressed patients from REM sleep also produced an antidepressant effect, although the onset of action appeared slower.

Although the effects of sleep deprivation are striking, they are short-lived. Only about 12% of those who respond clinically to sleep deprivation show continued improvement. The remainder show a depressive relapse following sleep the night after sleep deprivation. In some subjects, a short day-time nap is sufficient to reinstate depression. However, concomitant antidepressant treatment can help delay or prevent relapse of depression in about 25% of responders. It is also worth noting that manic switches are not uncommon following sleep deprivation, particularly in patients with bipolar depression.

The mechanism by which sleep deprivation produces antidepressant effects is unknown, but it is likely to be of great theoretical and clinical importance. Current hypotheses include a depressogenic substance which is secreted during sleep, and the build up of a hypothetical sleepiness process (process S) which has euphorogenic properties.[15]

Biochemistry and the pathophysiology of depression

Depressive disorders have a complex aetiology.[16,17] Important factors include genetic vulnerability, childhood difficulties, personality attributes, recent stressful life events and levels of social support (Table 5). Whatever the aetiological factors, it seems reasonable to assume that the clinical manifestations of depression are mediated ultimately through changes in brain neurochemistry. Biochemical investigations in depressed patients have focused on the monoamine neurotransmitters, particularly noradrenaline and 5-HT, because most antidepressant drugs produce prominent effects on these neurotransmitter pathways. Of course, the actions of antidepressant

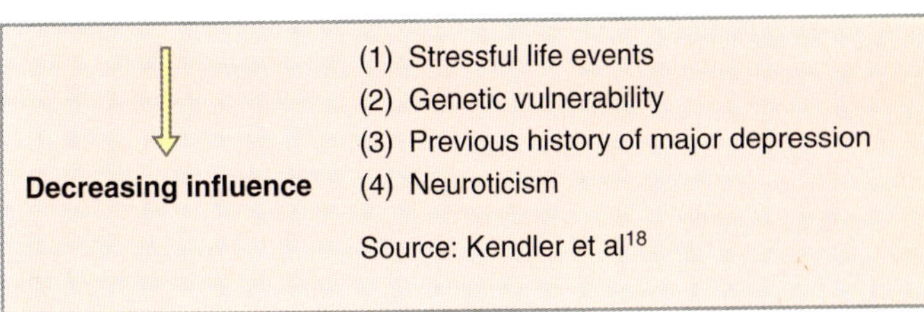

Table 5
Factors predicting liability to depression in women.

drugs may not reverse the biochemical causes of depression; monoamines, however, play an important role in mediating adaptive responses to stress, and depressive disorders could be viewed as failure of these adaptive responses.

Methodological limitations

A major problem in understanding the biochemical basis of depression is that, until recently, investigations of the living human brain have not been technically feasible. Accordingly various indirect methods have been employed to assess neurotransmitter function, including:

- Plasma levels of neurotransmitters and their precursors
- Neurotransmitter receptor binding on blood cells
- Neuroendocrine challenge tests
- Cerebrospinal fluid (CSF) sampling of neurotransmitters and their metabolites
- Post-mortem brain studies of neurotransmitters and their receptors

Despite much investigation, there is still little certain knowledge about how abnormalities in neurotransmitter function may contribute to the pathophysiology of depressive disorders. Some of the more reliably elicited abnormalities in 5-HT, noradrenaline, dopamine and acetylcholine function will be outlined below (Table 6).

5-HT abnormalities

Most studies have found that plasma levels of the 5-HT precursor tryptophan are low in depressed patients. The availability of tryptophan to the brain plays a critical role in regulating brain 5-HT synthesis and therefore lowered levels of plasma tryptophan might be associated with decreased brain 5-HT function. In general, however, the lowering of plasma tryptophan is modest and therefore unlikely to compromise brain 5-HT function to a clinically significant extent.

5-HT	(1) ↓ Plasma tryptophan
	(2) ↓ Prolactin release to 5-HT challenge
	(3) ↑ 5-HT$_2$ receptors in cortex
Noradrenaline	(1) ↓ Growth hormone response to noradrenaline challenge
	(2) ↓ Suppression by clonidine of REM sleep
Dopamine	(1) ↓ HVA in CSF
Acetylcholine	(1) ↑ Growth hormone response to pyridostigmine
	(2) ↑ REM sleep onset to cholinergic challenge

Table 6
Some neurochemical abnormalities found in depressed patients.

The increase in plasma prolactin following challenge with 5-HT-promoting drugs is lowered in depressed patients. This neuroendocrine abnormality is found fairly reliably following challenge with drugs that facilitate the presynaptic release of 5-HT, for example tryptophan or the 5-HT-releasing agent fenfluramine. However endocrine responses to drugs acting at postsynaptic 5-HT receptors are not consistently altered in depressed subjects. This suggests that impaired prolactin responses to 5-HT challenge in depression are attributable to a deficit in presynaptic 5-HT pathways.

There is little evidence that the concentration of 5-HT or its metabolite, 5-hydroxyindolacetic acid (5-HIAA), is lowered in the CSF in a broad range of depressed patients. However, a subgroup of depressed patients who have made suicide attempts may have low CSF 5-HIAA. Interestingly, this abnormality may cut across diagnostic boundaries and is found, for example, in patients with schizophrenia and some with personality disorders who tend to behave in an aggressive way towards themselves or others. Despite this, post-mortem studies have not found reliable changes in 5-HT or 5-HIAA in suicide victims, many of whom would probably have suffered from severe depression. There are reports that the binding of a subtype of postsynaptic 5-HT receptor, the 5-HT$_2$ receptor, may be increased in depressed patients and suicide victims. However, this abnormality has not been consistently replicated.

Noradrenaline

There is fairly reliable evidence that the growth hormone response to the noradrenaline re-uptake inhibitor desipramine and the noradrenaline receptor agonist clonidine is blunted in patients with more severe forms of depression. Clonidine acts directly on postsynaptic α_2-adrenoceptors in the hypothalamus and therefore the blunted growth hormone response in depressed patients suggests a decreased responsivity of post-synaptic α_2-adrenoceptors in this brain region.

There is little consistent evidence for changes in levels of nor-adrenaline or its metabolites in the CSF of depressed patients. Similarly, there are no reproducible changes in brain nor-adrenaline concentrations in post-mortem studies of depressed patients. It is, however, possible that both patients dying while depressed and suicide victims may have lowered binding of α_1-adrenoceptors in some brain regions.

Dopamine

The function of dopamine in depression has been less studied than that of 5-HT or noradrenaline. The CSF levels of the dopamine metabolite, homovanillic acid (HVA) have been reported to be low in several studies of depressed patients. On the other hand no consistent changes have been found in post-mortem studies of brain dopamine and HVA levels. Overall dopamine-mediated neuroendocrine responses seem to be unchanged in depressed patients.

Acetylcholine

Acetylcholine has been less studied in depression than the monoamines. However it has been proposed that depression may be characterized by a relative imbalance of acetylcholine and noradrenaline such that acetylcholine function is increased while that of noradrenaline is decreased. This hypothesis is supported by the pharmacological effects of cholinergic agents in normal subjects. For example, anticholinesterases tend to produce depression while muscarinic antagonists such as atropine can cause euphoria.

Limited neuroendocrine data suggest that endocrine responses to cholinergic challenge are enhanced in depressed patients. For example, the growth hormone response to the anti-cholinesterase inhibitor pyridostigmine is exaggerated in depressed patients, suggesting that acetylcholine function may be increased.[19] Of great interest, in view of the decrease in REM sleep latency seen in depression, is the finding that cholinergic induction of REM sleep is facilitated in depressed subjects. Increased sensitivity of muscarinic cholinergic receptors provides a plausible explanation for the decreased REM sleep latency seen in many depressed patients (see below).

Biochemistry and impaired sleep in depression

Because impaired sleep is so common in depression, it is interesting to explore whether or not any of the abnormalities in sleep architecture and continuity can be explained by the hypothesized changes in brain monoamine and acetylcholine function in depression.[20]

Sleep continuity

As noted earlier, decreases in brain 5-HT function cause insomnia and therefore lowered 5-HT neurotransmission might account for decreased total sleep time. However, it is important to note that the effect of 5-HT lesioning on sleep in animals is rather temporary and over several days recovery of sleep occurs . In addition, acute and chronic administration of selective 5-HT re-uptake inhibitors can also cause sleep disruption.[9] It is therefore difficult to equate insomnia in a simple way with lowered brain 5-HT function. In general, reductions in noradrenaline neurotransmission cause increased sleep. Therefore lowered brain noradrenergic function cannot provide a straightforward explanation of the sleep impairment seen in depressed patients.

REM sleep

It is indeed possible to correlate the postulated changes in brain neurochemistry in depression with changes in REM sleep. It is well established that muscarinic cholinergic pathways play an important role in generating REM sleep, and there is evidence from both sleep and neuroendocrine studies that depressed patients may have supersensitive muscarinic receptors (see above). Accordingly, increased muscarinic receptor sensitivity provides a plausible explanation for the decrease in REM latency seen in depression.

Noradrenergic α_2-adrenoceptors are also involved in the regulation of REM sleep, although, somewhat confusingly, both the α_2-adrenoceptor agonist clonidine and the α_2-adrenoceptor antagonist idazoxan decrease REM sleep. In depressed patients the ability of clonidine to suppress REM sleep is significantly less than that of controls.[21] This suggests a subsensitivity of α_2-adrenoceptors which is consistent with the impaired growth hormone response to clonidine seen in depression. Accordingly, subsensitivity of α_2-adrenoceptors may be involved in the disorders of REM sleep seen in depressed patients.

5-HT pathways are also involved in the regulation of REM sleep. It has previously been noted that selective 5-HT re-uptake inhibitors decrease REM sleep and increase REM sleep latency, but effects of 5-HT receptor antagonists are less consistent. It is, however, possible to lower brain 5-HT function by a relatively simple dietary manipulation in which subjects are given an amino acid load which acutely decreases the availability of tryptophan to the brain. In healthy subjects, this procedure significantly shortens REM latency. It is therefore possible that decreased brain 5-HT neurotransmission may play a role in the decreased REM sleep latency seen in depression.

Slow wave sleep

Depressed patients also exhibit decreased slow wave sleep but this is difficult to account for in terms of lowered monoamine function. For example, administration of selective 5-HT_2 receptor antagonists to healthy subjects produces a large and enduring increase in slow wave sleep. These data make it unlikely that lowered 5-HT function can underlie the decrease in slow wave sleep seen in depressed patients.

Antidepressant drugs and sleep

Antidepressant drugs can produce striking changes in both the subjective experience of sleep and in sleep architecture. For the most part, these changes are explicable in terms of the pharmacological effects of the different classes of compounds (Table 7).

Pharmacology of antidepressant drugs[16]

Tricyclic antidepressants (TCAs)

In general TCAs inhibit the re-uptake of noradrenaline and, to a somewhat lesser extent, 5-HT. The exception to this is clomipramine which potently inhibits the re-uptake of 5-HT and, through its metabolite desmethylimipramine, that of noradrenaline as well. The ability to inhibit noradrenaline and 5-HT re-uptake probably underlies the antidepressant effect of TCAs.

In addition TCAs possess antagonist properties at various postsynaptic neurotransmitter receptors. These effects are more pronounced in tertiary amine derivatives such as

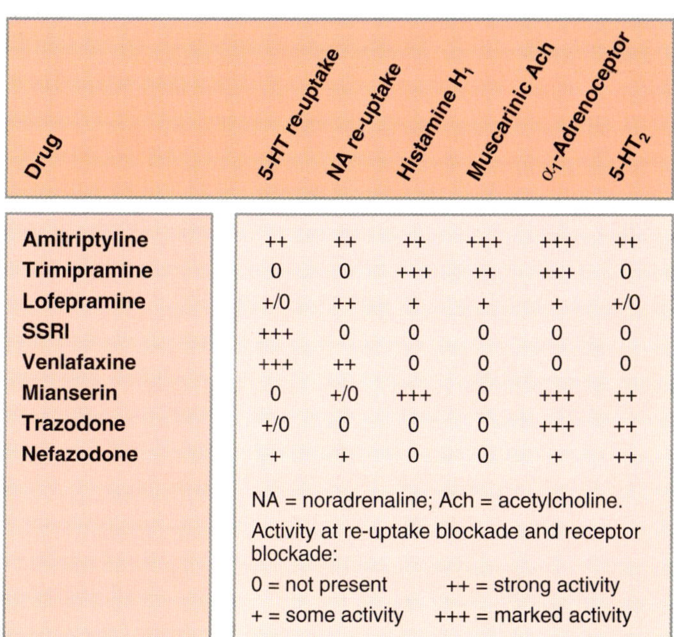

Drug	5-HT re-uptake	NA re-uptake	Histamine H_1	Muscarinic Ach	α_1-Adrenoceptor	5-HT$_2$
Amitriptyline	++	++	++	+++	+++	++
Trimipramine	0	0	+++	++	+++	0
Lofepramine	+/0	++	+	+	+	+/0
SSRI	+++	0	0	0	0	0
Venlafaxine	+++	++	0	0	0	0
Mianserin	0	+/0	+++	0	+++	++
Trazodone	+/0	0	0	0	+++	++
Nefazodone	+	+	0	0	+	++

NA = noradrenaline; Ach = acetylcholine.
Activity at re-uptake blockade and receptor blockade:
0 = not present   ++ = strong activity
+ = some activity   +++ = marked activity

Table 7
Activity of antidepressant drugs to inhibit monoamine re-uptake and block neurotransmitter receptors.

amitriptyline than in secondary amines such as nortriptyline. They include effects such as:

- α_1-Adrenoceptor blockade
- Muscarinic cholinergic receptor blockade
- Histamine H_1-receptor blockade
- 5-HT$_2$ receptor blockade

These receptor antagonist effects can account for most of the side effects of TCAs (Table 8) and for many of their effects on sleep and sleep architecture.

Pharmacological action	Adverse effect
Muscarinic receptor blockade (anticholinergic)	Dry mouth, tachycardia, constipation, urinary retention, glaucoma, cognitive impairment
α_1-Adrenoceptor blockade	Drowsiness, postural hypotension, sexual dysfunction, cognitive impairment
Histamine H_1-receptor blockade	Drowsiness, weight gain
5-HT$_2$ receptor blockade	Weight gain
Membrane-stabilizing properties	Cardiac arrhythmias

Table 8
Some adverse effects of tricyclic antidepressants.

The TCA lofepramine deserves a special mention because, although it is a tertiary amine, it is a fairly selective inhibitor of noradrenaline re-uptake and is relatively free from sedative and anticholinergic side-effects. In addition it lacks the toxicity in overdose associated with conventional TCAs.

Monoamine oxidase inhibitors (MAOIs)

These inactivate the enzymes that oxidize 5-HT, noradrenaline, dopamine, tyramine and other amines. There are two forms of MAO encoded by separate genes. In general MAO-A metabolizes intraneuronal noradrenaline and 5-HT, while both MAO-A and MAO-B metabolize dopamine and tyramine. The practical importance of this is that drugs which inhibit both MAO-A and MAO-B, such as tranylcypromine, phenelzine and isocarboxazid, can give rise to serious hypertensive interactions with tyramine-containing foodstuffs (the *cheese* reaction).

In contrast to conventional MAOIs, moclobemide binds reversibly and selectively to MAO-A. It is therefore relatively free from tyramine reactions but retains antidepressant activity. Interestingly, treatment with both conventional MAOIs and moclobemide can give rise to complaints of insomnia.

Selective serotonin re-uptake inhibitors (SSRIs)

The SSRIs include: citalopram, fluoxetine, fluvoxamine, paroxetine and sertraline. The acute pharmacological effect of all these compounds is essentially confined to blockade of 5-HT re-uptake. None of them has an appreciable affinity for the noradrenaline re-uptake site and present data suggest that they have a very low affinity for other neurotransmitter receptors.

The SSRIs have a side-effect profile that is distinct from that of TCAs and encompasses mainly gastrointestinal and central effects (Table 9). The SSRIs can often cause insomnia, but day-time somnolence can also be a problem. Sexual dysfunction, notably anorgasmia, is also relatively common. In contrast to conventional TCAs, SSRIs (with the possible exception of citalopram) are relatively free from toxicity in overdose, which is an important consideration in the treatment of some depressed patients.

Gastrointestinal	Nausea, anorexia, dry mouth, diarrhoea, dyspepsia, weight loss
Central nervous system	Headache, insomnia, dizziness, anxiety, fatigue, tremor, somnolence, extrapyramidal reactions
Other	Sweating, delayed orgasm/anorgasmia, hyponatraemia

Table 9
Some adverse effects of selective serotonin re-uptake inhibitors.

Venlafaxine

Venlafaxine is a phenylethylamine derivative which produces a potent blockade of both 5-HT and noradrenaline re-uptake. In this respect the pharmacological properties of venlafaxine resemble those of clomipramine. However, unlike clomipramine and other TCAs, venlafaxine has little affinity for other neurotransmitter receptor sites and therefore lacks anticholinergic and sedative properties. Venlafaxine has been classified a selective serotonin and noradrenaline re-uptake inhibitor (SNRI).

The adverse effect profile of venlafaxine resembles that of SSRIs with the most common adverse events being nausea, headache, dizziness, somnolence, insomnia and sexual dysfunction. An infrequent side-effect of venlafaxine is a dose-related increase in blood pressure. This may be attributable to facilitation of noradrenergic neurotransmission in the absence of postsynaptic α_1-adrenoceptor blockade.

Mianserin

Mianserin is a quadricyclic compound with complex pharmacological actions. It has weak noradrenaline re-uptake inhibiting effects and is a potent antagonist at 5-HT_2 receptors. Mianserin is also a competitive antagonist at histamine H_1 receptors and α_1- and α_2-adrenoceptors. It is not a muscarinic antagonist and is not cardiotoxic. These pharmacological properties give mianserin a sedating profile but it is not anticholinergic and lacks toxicity in overdose.

The main adverse effects of mianserin are drowsiness and dizziness. During longer-term treatment, weight gain can be problematic. The most serious adverse effect of mianserin is the rare appearance of leucopenia which may progress to agranulocytosis. It is therefore recommended that a blood count be obtained prior to initiation of mianserin treatment and that white cell counts be monitored monthly for 3 months after treatment has started.

Trazodone

Trazodone is a triazalopyridine derivative with complex actions on 5-HT pathways. Studies in vitro suggest that trazodone has weak 5-HT re-uptake inhibiting properties but during clinical treatment it does not significantly lower platelet 5-HT content, arguing against substantial 5-HT re-uptake blocking properties in vivo. Trazodone also has antagonist actions at 5-HT_2 receptors, but is metabolized to a 5-HT_2 receptor agonist, m-chlorophenylpiperazine (mCPP). The precise balance of effects on 5-HT receptors during trazodone treatment is therefore difficult to determine and may depend on the relative levels of parent compound and metabolite. Trazodone is an effective α_1-adrenoceptor antagonist which gives it a sedating profile in clinical use.

The major unwanted effect of trazodone is excessive drowsiness. Nausea and dizziness can also occur. Trazodone is less cardiotoxic than conventional TCAs, but there are reports that cardiac arrhythmias may be worsened in patients with cardiac disease. The most serious side effect of trazodone is priapism, which is seen rarely (about 1 in 6000 male patients). Treatment with noradrenergic agonists or even surgical decompression may be needed.

Nefazodone

Nefazodone is related to trazodone but lacks α_1-adrenoceptor antagonist properties. It is therefore not sedating. It has moderate 5-HT re-uptake inhibiting properties and is also a 5-HT_2 receptor antagonist. Nefazodone is metabolized to hydroxynefazodone whose clinical properties resemble those of the parent compound. It also metabolized to the 5-HT_2 receptor agonist mCPP, but during repeated treatment the 5-HT_2 receptor antagonist properties of nefazodone and hydroxynefazodone probably prevent expression of the pharmacological effects of mCPP.[22]

The use of nefazodone is associated with headache, dizziness, somnolence and nausea. It is less likely than SSRIs to cause insomnia and sexual dysfunction. Nefazodone is less cardio-toxic than conventional TCAs and therefore is likely to be safer in overdose.

Bupropion[23]

Bupropion is marketed for the treatment of depression in the USA but not in Europe. It is a unicyclic compound whose pharmacological properties are not well characterized. It may, however, have some activity as a dopamine and noradrenaline re-uptake inhibitor. Bupropion has activating properties and early in treatment can cause restlessness and insomnia. However, it does not cause significant sexual dysfunction. Bupropion is associated with an increased risk of seizures, particularly where the dose exceeds 450 mg daily.

Antidepressant drugs and sleep

In broad terms it is possible to derive the effects of antidepressant drugs on sleep from their pharmacological properties.[8] From what is known about the neurochemistry of sleep we would predict:

- Drugs that block the re-uptake of 5-HT or noradrenaline or both should lower REM sleep and increase REM latency
- Drugs that block muscarinic cholinergic receptors should decrease REM latency and REM sleep
- Drugs that have significant 5-HT_2 receptor antagonist properties should increase slow wave sleep
- Drugs that have prominent α_1-adrenoceptor or histamine H_1-receptor antagonist properties should increase sleep and sleep continuity
- Drugs that potentiate 5-HT and noradrenaline function in the absence of α_1-adrenoceptor or histamine H_1-receptor antagonist effects should decrease sleep and sleep continuity

The effects of antidepressant drugs on sleep have been studied in both healthy volunteers and depressed patients, but it is quite possible that the effects of drugs on the sleep of these two populations might differ. For example, underlying monoamine function may be abnormal in depression and the response to drugs acting on monoamine pathways could therefore be modified. In addition, if antidepressant drugs relieve the underlying depressive state, changes in sleep may then reflect both direct pharmacological effects of drug treatment and the consequences of clinical recovery.

REM sleep

The majority of antidepressant drugs decrease REM sleep and increase REM latency in both healthy subjects and depressed patients (Table 10). Of the TCAs, clomipramine produces the most profound suppression of REM sleep, although relatively selective noradrenaline re-uptake inhibitors such as desipramine, lofepramine and maprotiline produce this effect as well. Interestingly, trimipramine does not alter REM sleep but its ability to block the re-uptake of noradrenaline and 5-HT is weak. The ability of TCAs to inhibit REM sleep persists throughout repeated treatment, although some lessening of the degree of REM suppression is apparent in longer-term studies.[24]

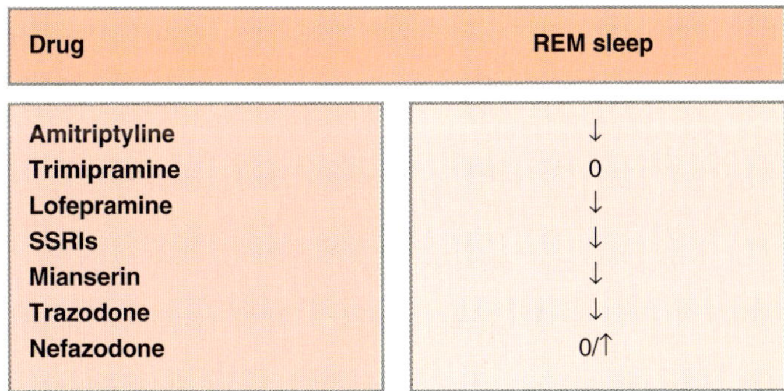

Drug	REM sleep
Amitriptyline	↓
Trimipramine	0
Lofepramine	↓
SSRIs	↓
Mianserin	↓
Trazodone	↓
Nefazodone	0/↑

Table 10
Effect of antidepressant drugs on REM sleep.

REM sleep is also diminished following treatment with conventional MAOIs such as phenelzine, but this effect is usually only apparent after several days' treatment. The effect of moclobemide on REM sleep is somewhat contradictory with both increases and decreases in REM sleep being reported.

The SSRIs also reliably decrease REM sleep following both acute and chronic administration in both patients and healthy subjects. The effect of mianserin is somewhat contradictory with one study finding no change in REM sleep in depressed patients although there was an increase in REM latency. In contrast, in healthy subjects mianserin administration did lower REM sleep. Most studies have found that trazodone decreases REM sleep and increases REM latency.[8]

The effects of nefazodone on REM sleep are not completely resolved but it seems fairly clear that it does not lower REM sleep or REM latency. In a single-dose, placebo-controlled study, Ware et al[25] found that nefazodone increased REM sleep but trazodone lowered it. On the other hand, depressed patients treated with chronic nefazodone did not show significant changes in REM sleep.[26] Similarly a recent 16-day placebo-controlled study in healthy subjects found no change in REM sleep time with nefazodone but a substantial decrease with paroxetine (Figure 9).[27]

Why nefazodone should not lower REM sleep when trazodone does is not clear. Nefazodone has less antagonist activity at α_1-adrenoceptors than trazodone but because α_1-adrenoceptor blockade appears to increase REM sleep,[5,6] this is unlikely to explain the different actions of the two drugs. Interestingly, bupropion treatment of depressed patients produced a significant increase in REM sleep.[28] Taken together, the findings with bupropion and nefazodone suggest that the ability to decrease REM sleep is not a requirement for a drug to possess antidepressant activity.

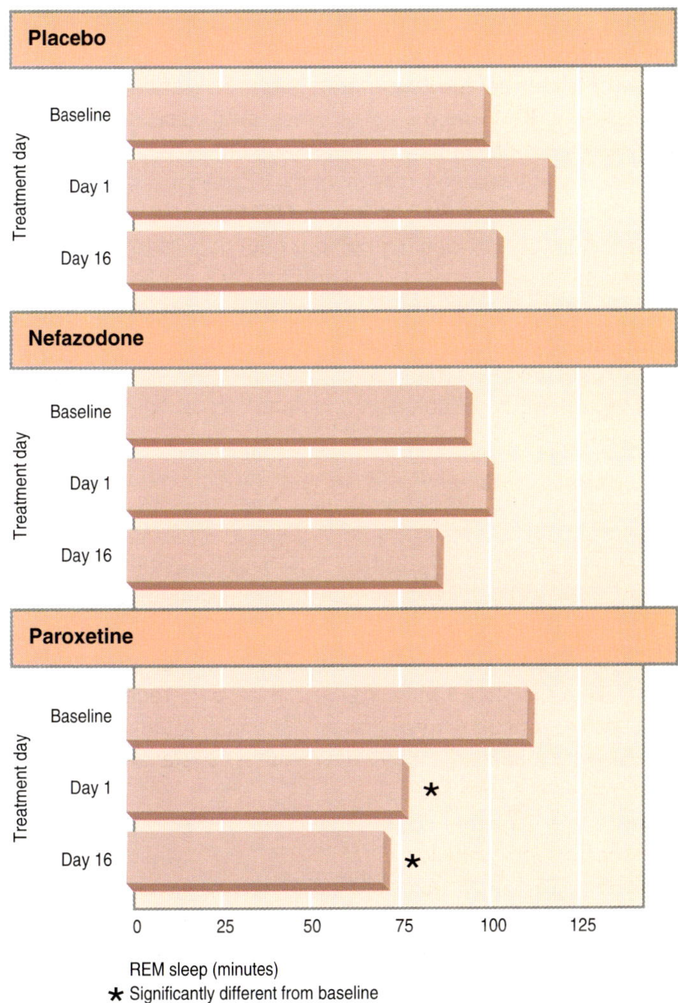

Figure 9

Effect of paroxetine and nefazodone treatment on REM sleep time in healthy subjects (denotes significantly less than baseline).*

Slow wave sleep

The effects of antidepressant drugs on slow wave sleep are quite variable but as expected those drugs that have potent 5-HT$_2$ receptor antagonist properties such as amitriptyline, mianserin and trazodone are reported to prolong the duration of slow wave sleep in either depressed patients or healthy subjects (Table 11). Assessment of the effect of antidepressants on slow wave sleep in depressed subjects is complicated by the fact that in some patients with a poor prognosis this stage of sleep remains diminished even after long-term treatment and clinical recovery.[13,14] In these circumstances slow wave sleep may be relatively refractory to pharmacological manipulation.

Drug	Slow wave sleep
Amitriptyline	↑
Trimipramine	0
Lofepramine	0
SSRIs	0/↓
Mianserin	↑
Trazodone	↑
Nefazodone	0

Table 11
Effect of antidepressant drugs on slow wave sleep.

In healthy volunteers SSRIs in single doses do not generally alter slow wave sleep. In depressed patients fluoxetine and fluvoxamine can decrease slow wave sleep, perhaps through indirect activation of 5-HT$_2$ receptors.[8] Although nefazodone has significant 5-HT$_2$ receptor antagonist properties, neither acute nor repeated administration to healthy subjects alters slow wave sleep.[8,27] Perhaps in this case the effect of 5-HT re-uptake blockade and 5-HT$_2$ receptor antagonism balance each other so that there is no net change in overall neurotransmission at 5-HT$_2$ receptors.

Sleep continuity

As noted earlier the complaint of poor sleep in depression is usually accompanied by objective evidence of poor sleep continuity characterized by frequent awakenings and overall lowered sleep efficiency. In addition, depressed patients often take a long time to fall asleep and show a prolonged latency to sleep on the sleep EEG. Antidepressants produce differing effects on measures of sleep continuity (Table 12), although resolution of the depressive disorder is usually accompanied by improvement in sleep continuity.

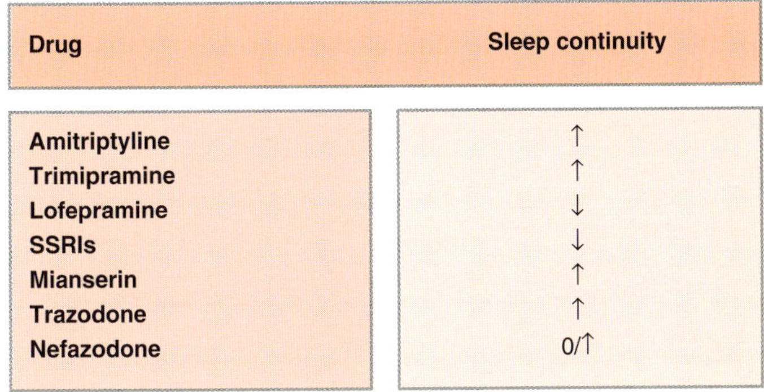

Drug	Sleep continuity
Amitriptyline	↑
Trimipramine	↑
Lofepramine	↓
SSRIs	↓
Mianserin	↑
Trazodone	↑
Nefazodone	0/↑

Table 12
Effect of antidepressant drugs on sleep continuity.

The TCAs, particularly the more sedating tertiary amines such as amitriptyline and trimipramine, are experienced as sedating and improve sleep continuity in both healthy subjects and depressed patients. In contrast lofepramine, which lacks significant sedating properties, decreases actual sleep time in healthy volunteers.[29] This is of interest because insomnia is a recognized adverse effect of lofepramine in clinical practice.[30] On the other hand, if sufficient time is given for clinical recovery, improvements can be seen in sleep continuity in depressed patients following longer-term treatment with non-sedating secondary TCAs such as desipramine.[24]

Insomnia is a frequent side effect of conventional MAOIs, particularly phenelzine and tranylcypromine.[16] For example, phenelzine lowers total sleep time in depressed patients. Insomnia is also reported as an adverse effect of moclobemide although it seems less problematic than with conventional MAOIs.[16] However, after repeated treatment in depressed patients moclobemide improved measures of sleep continuity, presumably through facilitating clinical recovery.[31]

SSRIs generally exhibit alerting effects and so are liable to impair sleep. In healthy volunteers, acute treatment with SSRIs lowers total sleep time, increases wakefulness and decreases sleep efficiency.[9] A 16-day course of paroxetine in healthy subjects produced a sustained increase in wake time and impaired sleep efficiency (Figure 10).[27] In depressed patients SSRIs can also produce impairments in sleep continuity that persist during longer-term treatment.[8,24] This may not be reported spontaneously, perhaps because the underlying improvement in mood may influence how insomnia is experienced by the patient.

Mianserin and trazodone are both sedating drugs which increase sleep continuity in depression. Nefazodone is of interest because although it is not sedating it may increase actual sleep time and sleep continuity in depressed patients and in some groups of healthy subjects.[8] It may, however, be hard to demonstrate improvement in sleep continuity measures in young healthy subjects because their baseline sleep efficiency is sufficiently high (above 90%) to make it difficult to obtain

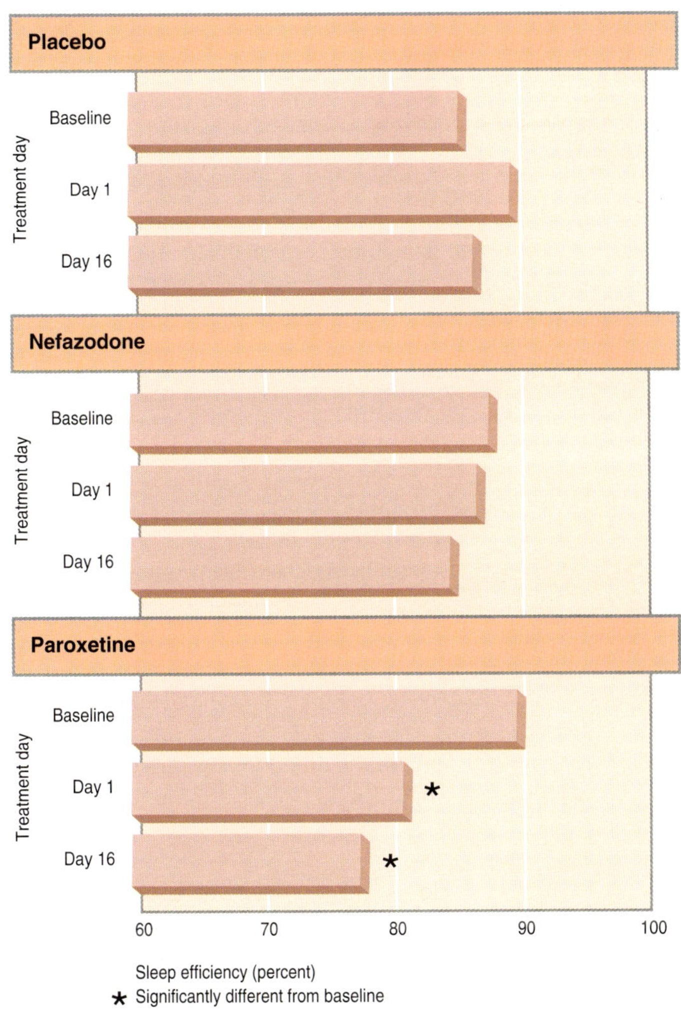

Figure 10

Effect of paroxetine and nefazodone treatment on sleep efficiency. (denotes significantly less than baseline).*

further improvement. For example, 16-days' treatment with nefazodone did not have a significant effect on sleep efficiency in a group of young male volunteers.[27]

During clinical treatment in depressed patients nefazodone is unlikely to cause insomnia. For example, in controlled studies the incidence of insomnia with nefazodone appeared no higher than that seen with placebo, in contrast to the subjective impairment of sleep caused by fluoxetine (Table 13).[32]

	Nefazodone (n=1022)	Fluoxetine (n=97)	Imipramine (n=367)
Insomnia	0.1	14.8*	0.4
Somnolence	5.8*	10.9*	12.0*
	*Significantly greater than placebo		

Table 13
Placebo-adjusted incidence (%) of patient-rated insomia and somnolence for nefazodone, fluoxetine and imipramine (data taken from reference[32]).

Clinical management of sleep disorders in depression

Clinical assessment

Impaired sleep is an important feature of clinical depressive disorders and eliciting sleep difficulties is part of the standard assessment of depression. As discussed earlier, patients may have a variety of abnormalities in initiation and maintenance of sleep and the nature of these should be clarified. A number of other issues are also worth discussing with the patient:

- What is your sleep like normally? Did your sleep problem begin only when you became depressed?
- How troublesome is poor sleep for you? Does it really bother you?
- How do you deal with insomnia? Do you try to prevent it and what do you do when it happens?
- Do you take daytime naps to catch up on sleep

Sleep hygiene during non-pharmacological treatment

Many patients with milder or transient depressive states can be managed with simple psychological techniques such as problem solving. In addition, more structured psychotherapies such as cognitive therapy may also be employed. It is of interest to note, however, that patients with clear abnormalities in sleep architecture may not respond well to cognitive therapy as a sole treatment.[33] Where patients do respond to psychological approaches some improvement in sleep continuity may be expected with clinical recovery. However, simple advice may also benefit the sleep disturbance (see page 10 – Sleep Hygiene).

Sleep disorder and suicide

It is also a standard part of the assessment of patients with depression to enquire about suicidal ideation. There appear to be significant clinical links between suicide and severe insomnia in the setting of depressive illness. For example, from a review of the literature, Teicher et al[34] noted that patients who eventually committed suicide often complained of severe insomnia which they found particularly troublesome. In the suicide study of Barraclough et al,[35] insomnia was the most prevalent overall symptom (76% of subjects) and 64% of suicide victims were taking hypnotic drugs.

The importance of insomnia in severe depression is clearly relevant to the use of psychotropic drugs. For example, in suicidal patients who are greatly troubled by insomnia it may be important to improve sleep early in treatment and not simply to wait until clinical remission occurs.

Choice of antidepressant

As seen earlier, there is now a wide range of antidepressant drugs available for the treatment of major depression. In the broad range of depressed patients these drugs appear of similar efficacy. The main distinction of clinical importance, therefore, is their adverse effect profile. This is particularly the case in primary care where patients are often striving to continue with their usual work and social activities.

Antidepressant drugs and sleep

While the effect of antidepressant drugs on sleep architecture is of interest, it is not clear how relevant this is to clinical outcome. We simply do not know, for example, the implications (if any) for the patient of taking a drug which suppresses REM sleep (for example, paroxetine), in comparison to one that does not (for example, nefazodone).

From the clinical viewpoint, therefore, the main distinction between the drugs is how they may affect the subjective sleep of the patient. As we have seen earlier this will relate mainly to measures of sleep continuity where increased continuity will be experienced as better sleep. Clearly, in the longer term the expectation is that the experience of sleep will improve anyway, as the depression remits. However, in the first few weeks of treatment the antidepressant is likely to have a direct impact on sleep through its pharmacological properties and this will affect how the patient perceives the drug treatment and, perhaps, how well the treatment is received.

Sedating antidepressants

As noted earlier drugs that have α_1-adrenoceptor antagonist properties and H_1-receptor antagonist properties are sedating and improve sleep. Such drugs include tertiary TCAs such as amitriptyline, clomipramine, dothiepin, doxepin, imipramine and trimipramine. Tertiary TCAs have two other properties important in their adverse effect profile, namely anticholinergic effects and cardiotoxicity in overdose.

Trazodone and mianserin lack anticholinergic properties and are safer in overdose than conventional TCAs. They are therefore useful alternatives to tertiary TCAs in patients where anticholinergic effects are contra-indicated or the risk of overdose is high and cannot be minimized. In addition, they are safer for patients who may have cardiovascular disease. The main problem with sedating antidepressants is the presence of

daytime sedation which may impair performance on some cognitive tasks.[36]

Non-sedating antidepressants

Secondary TCAs such as desipramine and nortriptyline are
much less sedating than tertiary TCAs. Lofepramine also
shares this profile. They retain, however, some anticholinergic
properties and, with the exception of lofepramine, are toxic in
overdose. Newer drugs such as the SSRIs and venlafaxine
generally lack sedative properties, although some patients

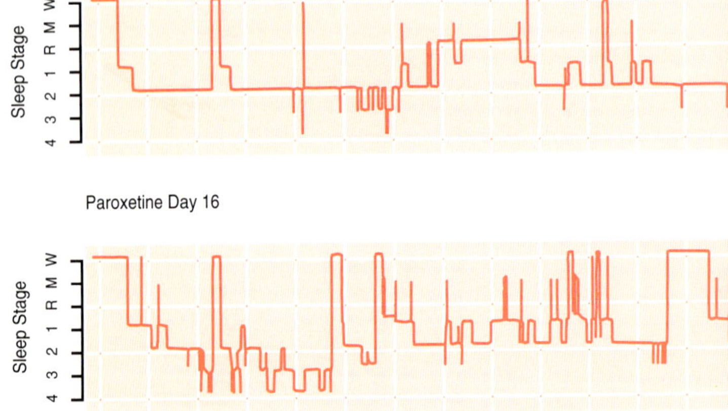

Figure 11
*Effect of 16 days' paroxetine treatment on the sleep hypnogram of a healthy
subject showing increased wake (W) and movement (M) time during the sleep
period.*

complain of daytime somnolence. In general, however, they seem less likely to impair daytime cognitive performance.[36] In addition, SSRIs and venlafaxine are not anticholinergic and are safer in overdose than conventional TCAs.

The problem with non-sedating antidepressants such as the SSRIs is that they can impair sleep (Figure 11). As noted above, sleep disruption may be tolerated poorly, particularly by more severely depressed patients. Clinical improvement is likely to improve sleep eventually but there is some evidence with SSRIs, for example, that the lowered sleep continuity can persist.

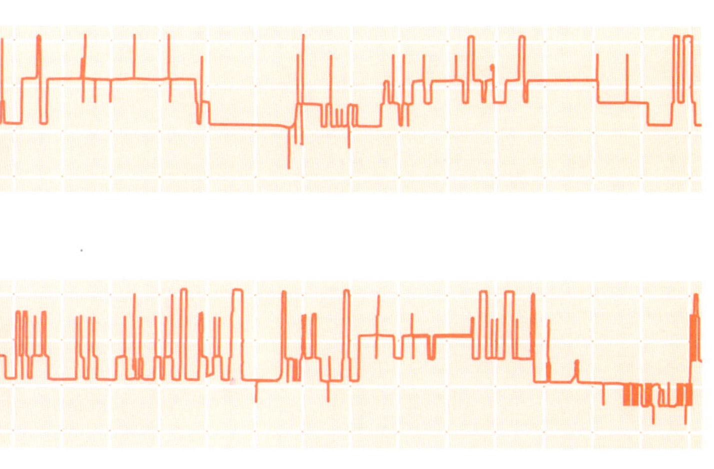

It is, of course, possible to treat sleep difficulties associated with drugs such as SSRIs and venlafaxine with short-acting benzodiazepines or small doses of trazodone. However, these approaches have their problems. For example, it is usually wise to avoid the initiation of benzodiazepine therapy where possible because it may be difficult to stop. Trazodone is probably less problematic in this respect but even low doses can cause daytime sedation. In contrast, nefazodone is less sedating than either trazodone or tertiary TCAs and does not appear to impair sleep (Figure 12).

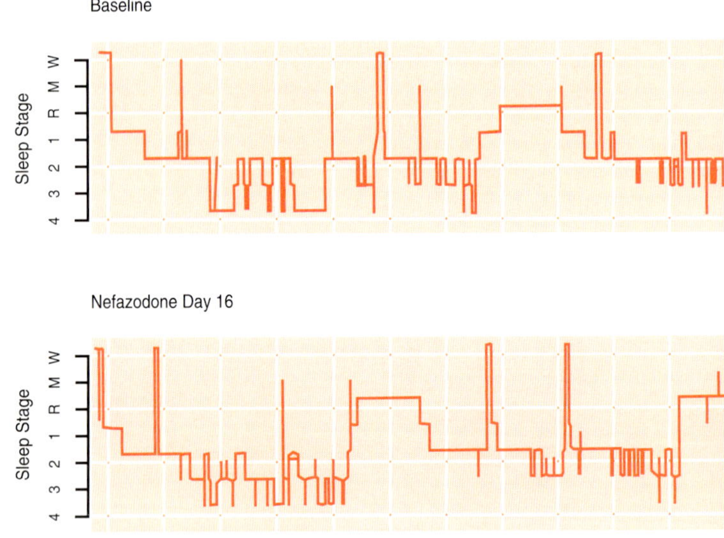

Figure 12
Effect of 16 days' nefazodone treatment on the sleep hypnogram of a healthy subject.

At present, therefore, there are several drugs that are suitable first-line agents for the treatment of major depression. Drug prescription is part of a complex clinical decision-making process which will include factors such as previous treatment response, tolerance of a particular adverse effect profile and cost. Factors such as sleep disturbance will also influence choice of antidepressant and attention to sleep impairment in patients troubled by poor sleep is likely to improve the therapeutic effect of drug treatment.

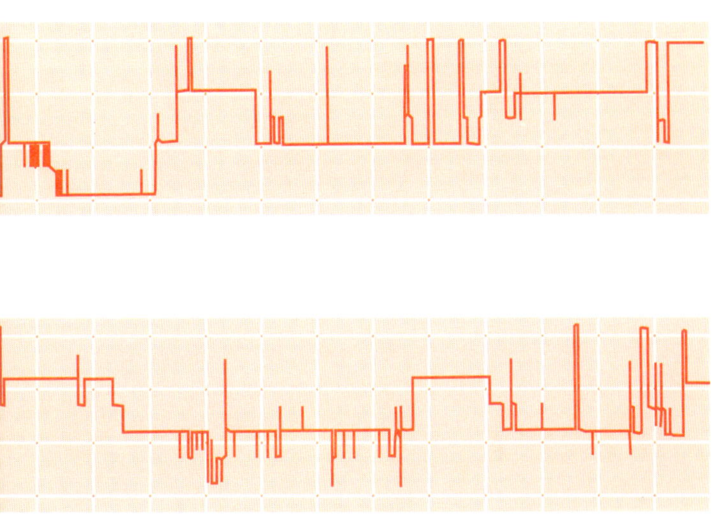

References

1   Idzikowski C and James R (1991) Sleep. In: *Serotonin, Sleep and Mental Disorder* (eds. C Idzikowski and PJ Cowen), pp. 23–32. Petersfield: Wrightson.

2   Horne J (1988) *Why we sleep*. Oxford: Oxford University Press.

3   Lasagna L (1995) Over-the-counter hypnotics and chronic insomnia in the elderly. *J Clin Psychopharmacol* **15**: 383–386.

4   American Psychiatric Association (1995) *Diagnostic and Statistical Manual of Mental Disorders* 4th edn, international version. Washington DC: American Psychiatric Press.

5   Parkes JD (1985) Pharmacology and sleep. In: *Sleep and its Disorders*, pp. 407–434. London: W B Saunders.

6   Sharpley AL and Idzikowski C (1991) Neurotransmitters and sleep. In: *Serotonin, Sleep and Mental Disorder* (eds. C Idzikowski and PJ Cowen), pp. 195-213. Petersfield: Wrightson.

7   Jacobs BL, Fornal CA and Wilkinson LO (1990) Neuro-physiologic and neurochemical studies of brain serotonergic neurones in behaving animals. In: *The Neuropharmacology of Serotonin* (eds. PM Whitaker-Azmitia and SJ Peroutka), pp. 260–268. New York: New York Academy of Science.

8   Sharpley AL and Cowen PJ (1995) Effect of pharmacologic treatments on the sleep of depressed patients. *Biol Psychiatry* **37**: 85–98.

9 Nicholson AN and Pascoe PA. (1991) Monoaminergic transmission and sleep in man. In: *Serotonin, Sleep and Mental Disorder* (eds. C Idzikowski and PJ Cowen), pp. 215–226. Petersfield: Wrightson.

10 Cianchetti C, Masala C, Mangoni A et al (1980) Suppression of REM and delta sleep by apomorphine in man: a dopamine mimetic effect. *Psychopharmacology* **67**: 61–65.

11 Hallstrom C (1994) Zopiclone. *Prescribers J* **34**: 115–118.

12 Styron W. (1990) *Darkness Visible.* London: Picador.

13 Kupfer DJ (1995) Sleep research in depressive illness: clinical implications – a tasting menu. *Biol Psychiatry* **38**: 391–403.

14 Kupfer DJ and Reynolds CF (1992) Sleep and affective disorders. In: *Handbook of Affective Disorders* (ed. ES Paykel), pp. 311–323. Edinburgh: Churchill Livingstone.

15 Wu JC and Bunney WE (1990) The biological basis of an antidepressant response to sleep deprivation and relapse: review and hypothesis. *Am J Psychiatry* **147**: 14–21.

16 Gelder MG, Gath DH, Mayou RA et al (1996) Mood disorders. In: *Oxford Textbook of Psychiatry*, pp. 197–245. Oxford: Oxford University Press.

17 Delgado PL, Price LH, Heninger GR et al. (1992) Neurochemistry. In: *Handbook of Affective Disorders* (ed. ES Paykel), pp. 219–253. Edinburgh: Churchill Livingstone.

18 Kendler KS, Kessler RC, Neale MC et al (1993) The prediction of major depression in women: toward an integrated etiologic model. *Am J Psychiatry* **150**: 1139–1148.

19 O'Keane V, O'Flynn K, Lucey J et al (1992) Pyridostigmine-induced growth hormone responses in healthy and depressed subjects: evidence for cholinergic supersensitivity in depression. *Psychol Med* **22**: 55–60.

20 Mendelson WB (1991) Neurotransmitters, sleep and affective disorder. In: *Serotonin, Sleep and Mental Disorder* (eds. C Idzikowski and PJ Cowen), pp. 277–288. Petersfield: Wrightson.

21 Schittecatte M, Garcia-Valentin J, Charles G et al (1995) Efficacy of the 'clonidine REM suppression test (CREST)' to separate patients with major depression from controls: a comparison with three currently proposed biological markers of depression. *J Affect Disord* **33**: 151–157.

22 Walsh AES and Cowen PJ (1994) Attenuation of the prolactin-stimulating and hypothermic effects of nefazodone following subacute treatment. *J Clin Psychopharmacol* **14**: 268–273.

23 Ascher JA, Cole JO, Colin JN et al (1995) Bupropion: a review of its mechanism of antidepressant activity. *J Clin Psychiatry* **56**: 395–401.

24 Kupfer DJ, Perel JM, Pollock BG et al (1991) Fluvoxamine versus desipramine: comparative polysomnographic effects. *Biol Psychiatry* **29**: 23–40.

25 Ware JC, Rose V and McBrayer R (1991) The effects of nefazodone, trazodone, buspirone and placebo on sleep and sleep related penile erections (NPT) in normal subjects. *Sleep Res* **20**: 91.

26 Armitage R, Rush AJ, Trivedi M et al (1994) The effects of nefazodone on sleep architecture in depression. *Neuropsychopharmacology* **10**: 123–127.

27 Sharpley AL, Williamson DJ, Attenburrow MEJ et al (1996) The effect of paroxetine and nefazodone on sleep: a placebo controlled trial. *Psychopharmacology* **126**: 50–54.

28 Nofzinger EA, Reynolds CF, Thase ME et al (1995) REM sleep enhancement by bupropion in depressed men. *Am J Psychiatry* **152**: 274–276.

29 Herdman JRE, Cowen PJ, Campling GM et al (1993) Effect of lofepramine on 5-HT function and sleep. *J Affect Disord* **29**: 63–72.

30 Lancaster SG and Gonzalez JP (1989) Lofepramine: a review of its pharmacodynamic and pharmacokinetic properties and therapeutic efficacy in depressive illness. *Drugs* **37:** 123–140.

31 Monti JM (1989) Effect of a reversible monoamine oxidase-A inhibitor (moclobemide) on sleep of depressed patients. *Br J Psychiatry* **155** (Suppl): 61–65.

32 Preskorn SH (1995) Comparison of the tolerability of bupropion, fluoxetine, imipramine, nefazodone, paroxetine, sertraline and venlafaxine. *J Clin Psychiatry* **56** (Suppl 6): 12–21.

33 Thase ME, Simons AD and Reynolds CF (1996) Abnormal electroencephalographic sleep profiles in major depression: association with response to cognitive behaviour therapy. *Arch Gen Psychiatry* **53**: 99–108.

34 Teicher MH, Glod CA and Cole JO (1993) Antidepressant drugs and the emergence of suicidal tendencies. *Drug Safety* **8**: 186–212.

35 Barraclough BM, Bunch J, Nelson B et al (1974) A hundred cases of suicide: clinical aspects. *Br J Psychiatry* **125**: 355–373.

36 Hale AS (1994) The importance of accidents in evaluating the cost of SSRIs: a review. *Int Clin Psychopharmacol* **9**: 195–201.

37 Whittington R and McTavish D (1995) Nefazodone: a review of its pharmacological properties and therapeutic potential in depressive illness. *Drugs* **49**: 1–22.

Index

Page numbers in italic refer to the illustrations